I0427963

Sugar Detox

Lose Weight, Feel Great, and Look Younger

Simon Roche

Finicky Inc.

New York

About me

FREE Bonus: [https://healthresultswealth.wordpress.com/ **]**
Motivational Coffee

Hi, my name is Simon Roche, Founder of "Finicky.us" and also the author to many entrepreneurial and self-help books.

I have seen that I was different since I was a kid. When other kids wanted to play, I wanted to be productive and better myself. Not to say that I didn't play on my free time, I just didn't play longer than I needed. I always set my expectations out of my reach and I truly hope that my readers do the same. I have visited many companies during my career and I can say that I have learned more than if I were to have worked for a company.

As a thank you for considering my book, I will provide you with one of my many experiences while visiting a friend at Google. My friend who was previously the "Strategic Partner Lead" at Google has had many accomplish through his career and no longer works at Google. We became friends in our marketing course and have still kept in contact.

He gave me a tip about the process of hiring people for my company. During the selection process, he weaves out many strong candidates. Why? Simply because they aren't smarter than me, the interviewer. He explains that if you want a good company, then you surround yourself with average brains that just want to get by. At Google, we don't want average, we want the smartest. Smart people hire smarter people and that's how Google is still on top of its industry. He stated, "I want to hire someone who is smarter than me, works better than me, and is more innovative than me. That way I will be happy when they take my position, as I move on to another chapter in my life"

Through my books, I will share many of my unique experiences and will provide you with mistakes that I have made myself as an entrepreneur.

Words from the Author

Before you start reading this book, I will need you to keep a thought in mind.

"To be able to sacrifice what you are, for who you will become"

In other words, if you put aside your excuses, you will get the results you have always wanted. It's time to make a decision. You can choose to stay the way you are or you can decide to take steps towards change.

No one is stopping you from where you want to go, the only person that is stopping you is YOU. Remind yourself every day of who you want to be, and remember to make the right decisions towards your goal. One way to keep your goals set is by checking up on yourself at the end of each week. Set a goal for 2 pounds each week, and by the end of the month you will have cut 8 pounds. Keep your short-term goals small so that it is achievable, but keep your long-term goals big, so that there is no ceiling towards your success.

Table of Contents

About me

Words from the Author

Introduction

Delving Deeper Into Sugar

The Bitter Truth about Sugar

The Devil Is In The Detail...

The Ultimate Sugar Detox Diet

Recipes

Don't Be Part Of The Statistic! (Conclusion)

Bonus from the Author

Preview of my book, 9 Powerful Habits

Sugar Detox Diet

Introduction

Every day when going about your daily activities, what's the first thing that catches your eye? For me, it is the fast rising number of obese and overweight kids as well as adults. The saddest part is that, this is what you can see from the outside, what about the maladies within the body that cannot be seen by the naked eye?

Diseases of civilization – obesity, hypertension, diabetes, cancer, stroke and the like are at an all-time high. What does this mean? If we don't do anything about this, most of us will not live long enough to see our grand kids! Can you even begin to fathom this?

Well, this is the reason why I was inspired to share with you, the number one culprit in fueling chronic illnesses – sugar, and what we need to do to cleanse our bodies and get back on the healthy living bandwagon.

Here, you are going to learn why it has been so hard to shake off your 'addiction' to sugar; to shed off those extra pounds; why you always seem to be losing a battery every time you try getting physical and how sugar is destroying your health and how to beat it once and for all!

Delving Deeper Into Sugar

Sugar is one of life's tasty little treats that most of us crave day in day out. Unfortunately we have become so hooked on sugar that doctors are warning that it is gradually turning into the new tobacco. According to a recent study in the UK, each of us takes an average of 15 teaspoon of sugar a day! Shocking, right?

But, exactly what is sugar?

Sugars are basically simple carbohydrates meaning they require very minimal digestion and thus are a very quick source of energy for your body. You will find sugar in fruits, milk products and foods with added artificial sugars such as sweets, candy and pastry.

An important point to note is that your body does not discern which sugar comes from where, that is, whether you eat sugar from candy or from fruit, it will be used by your body in the same way. However, sugar found in fruits, milk and other natural foods comes with nutrients such as vitamins and minerals, whereas those found in sweets, pastry and other artificially added sugars have very little, if any, nutritional value.

The different types of sugar

Sugar comes in many different forms though all the different forms come with a sweet flavor. The two main types of sugar are;

Sucrose – this type of sugar is made from fructose and glucose

Fructose – this type of sugar is found in fruit and honey

And we also have lactose from milk.

Syrups

Most syrups used are made from pure sucrose and are commonly used in the food manufacturing process to add great flavor and color. Golden syrup is made from the breaking down of two chain sucrose (disaccharides) to glucose and fructose through a process called inversion that prevents crystallization during its storage.

White sugar

This is purely made from sucrose that is derived from sugarcane and beets. There is no real difference between white sugar produced from sugarcane and that produced from sugar beets. However, some manufacturers produce crystals of different sizes which make us believe that white sugar with smaller crystals is sweeter than that with large crystals but this is only because smaller crystals dissolve faster.

Brown sugar

This is basically sucrose mixed with a bit of molasses that's responsible for its brown color and the rich flavor.

Artificial sweeteners

These are synthetic sugar substitutes but some are derived from natural foods such as fruit and vegetables. Artificial sweeteners are also referred to as intense sweeteners as they are many times sweeter than conventional sugar. The currently approved sweeteners are:

Aspartame

This sweetener is mostly used in candy, soda and dessert. It is between 180-200 times sweeter than regular white sugar.

Saccharin

This sweetener has a bitter almost metallic aftertaste. It is however not digested by the body and passes directly through your digestive tract. It is 400 times sweeter than regular white sugar.

Neotame

This sweetener is extremely sweet; it is 40 times as sweet as aspartame and 8000 times as sweet as regular white sugar. Very minute portions are used to sweeten and add flavor to foods.

Sucralose

This is 600 times sweeter than regular white sugar. It is very common in canned fruit, candy bars, breakfast bars and even soft drinks.

TIP:

1 gram of sugar has 4 calories. Women should not consume more than 100 calories from sugar and for men, not more than 150 calories in a day.

The Bitter Truth about Sugar

One of the major problems with sugar is its ability to masquerade into breakfast, lunch, dinner, dessert or even a snack especially if the food in question is processed. By just looking at a label, it is very hard to distinguish between natural sugars versus sugar that has been added.

You will be shocked to find out that many foods that are labeled 'healthy' at times contain shocking amounts fructose and added sugars that in most cases are in the form of high fructose corn syrup (HFCS). If you were to pick out the worst villain in sugars, it would be fructose.

For you to watch your sugar intake and remain healthy, you need to learn how to distinguish between added sugars versus natural food-based sugars. A good example is a small serving cup of fruit flavored yogurt which contains 19g of sugar, 12 g of which are added sugars while the same sized cup of plain, natural yogurt contains 7g of sugar from lactose, a natural sugar that is found in milk that doesn't cause much harm.

The 'low-fat' ideology is particularly harmful because when food manufacturers removed fat, they had to make up for this with truckloads of sugar. The thing is, when fat is removed from most foods, the result is unpalatable food and the only way to retain the flavor is to add more and more sugar.

The bitter truth is that healthy nutrition includes a good serving of healthy fats and sugar in fact is the number one driver of chronic inflammation that is directly linked to major health problems such as diabetes, heart disease, obesity, cancer and so on.

The simple truth is that when the food manufacturers substituted fat with sugar, they created an express smorgasbord of ready to order illnesses. These processed foods also contain other ingredients such as Trans fats, glyphosate, genetically engineered ingredients and artificial sweeteners; when added sugars are put in the equation, they act as the final nail on the coffin!

Understand that sugar by any other name is STILL SUGAR!

The reason why so many of us are taking an excess of sugar day in day out is that we are not even aware we are eating sugar 50% of the time. You have probably come across the terms maltose, maltodextin, dextrose and galactose. Added sugars masquerade in 74% of available processed foods under more than 60 'code names'

The instant 'high' we get right after eating sugar is one of the main reasons we turn to it when we are hungry, crave reward or comfort or at times of celebration. You may not think of yourself as having a sweet tooth but the amount of sugar you take unknowingly every single day might shock you. Breakfast cereal, soups bread, pasta, pasta sauce, ketchup and so on are laced with added sugars in names that we can't even pronounce.

But, is sugar all bad?

No! Sugar is not all bad news. Our bodies need some sugar to supply ready fuel to our muscles and to also keep our brains active. The problem is that most of our foods today are processed and have loads of added sugars which provide energy purely from calories and nothing else. Our bodies are thus forced to draw on essential nutrients from other foods in our diet to process the sugar and this can negatively affect our health and especially our immunity.

A high sugar intake causes your blood sugar levels to skyrocket, giving you an awesome high followed by an almost immediate crash slump that leaves you irritable, feeling tired and craving for more and more sugar. This vicious cycle contributes to weight gain and serious chronic illnesses stemming from chronic inflammation.

How much sugar can your body handle?

The main issue with sugar and artificial fructose in particular, is that your liver doesn't have much capacity to metabolize it. According to researchers, your body can safely metabolize approximately 6 teaspoons of added sugars every day but, the average person takes approximately 22 teaspoons of sugar every single day!

All the excess sugar that you consume is metabolized into body fat which leads to nearly all of the chronic illnesses that we struggle with every day such as:

- Hypertension
- Cancer
- Type 2 diabetes
- Dementia
- Cardiovascular diseases
- Metabolic syndrome

Why can't I stop drinking soda?

So many of us can't seem to resist the allure of drinking one more can of soda and this is not because you do not have a strong willpower! Nearly all soft drinks contain caffeine which is a mild diuretic causing you to urinate more. By doing this, you eliminate loss of water from your body. In addition, each can or bottle of soda contains about 55mg of salt.

When you take in salt and eliminate water, you get thirstier and thirstier. But first, the soda industry has to mask the salt in soda and the only way to do this is to kick-up the sugar content and the result is a very sweet and refreshing drink that you can't seem to get enough of especially when ice cold.

This is a very effective business strategy that's used by soda manufacturing giants to drive sales. Unfortunately, this business strategy is crippling customers health wise and slowly but effectively killing us. And what's more, sugar has been found to be eight times more addictive than cocaine! We will be looking at this further into the book and also look at how to fight off the cravings and eliminate processed sugars from your daily routine.

What's the connection between sugar and cancer?

Sugar, is a subject that is yet to be totally understood. Sometimes you will walk in hospitals and find cancer patients being served processed foods that have a high sugar content despite the fact that all science clearly points out that sugar literally feeds cancer.

The thing is cancer cells need food for them to thrive and this food in essence is glucose. When you consume carbohydrates, they are converted into glucose in your body but in order to starve cancer cells, you have to cut off its primary source of food – sugars that include all non-fruit and non-vegetable carbohydrates.

The World Health Organization released a report that predicts an increase in worldwide cancer rates by a whopping 57% in the next 20 years! This report also notes that half of all cancers can be avoided and prevented if healthy diets and exercise are implemented and if all the current medical knowledge is exercised.

The very simple truth is that by reducing processed food and sugar consumption, we will have won more than half the battle with cancer.

The Devil Is In The Detail...

The only way to preserve and protect your health is to know where added sugars hide so you can stay away from them. Here are some handy ways to spot all the hidden sugars;

- 'Diet foods' such as low fat foods more often than not contain extra sugars to improve their taste and to also add texture and bulk in the place of fat.
- A can of soda or soft drink contains no less than 7 teaspoons of sugar with diet soda being worse because it has additional artificial sweeteners that are digested very fast by your body.
- Savory foods such a soups, chips, corn puffs, readymade sauces and soups contain added sugar to give them a great final taste
- Natural sugar in some fruit such as Jazz, Fuji and Pink Lady apples has been increased through genetic modification to meet the needs of our sweet tooth.

Lean how to read labels correctly

Discover exactly how much sugar is in your food by making these simple checks:

- Check the food item's ingredients list for anything ending with 'ose' (fructose, glucose, lactose, sucrose, and maltose). Also look out for honey, molasses, agave and syrups like rice and corn syrup. The higher these items appear on the ingredients list, the more sugar the food item contains.

- Read the carbs as sugars on the nutrition section – this will include both the natural and added sugars. If it reads less than 5g per 100g, this means that the food item contains little sugar. However, if it contains more than 15g per 100g, the food items contains high sugar levels.

The hidden sugars

Dextrose, glucose, barley matt, molasses, beet sugar, white sugar, molasses, raw sugar, buttered syrup, fruit juice, cane juice crystals, caramel, date sugar, cane sugar, diastase, golden sugar, maltodextrin, high fructose corn syrup, yellow sugar, sorghum syrup, refiner's syrup, invert sugar, sorbitol, turbinado sugar, diastatic malt, dextran, fruit juice concentrate, ethyl syrup, maltol, carob syrup, corn syrup, mannitol, honey, glucose solids, corn syrup solids, sucrose, golden syrup.

- Beware of your substitutes. For example mannitol, sorbital and xylitol occur naturally in fruits ad plants in small amounts and are mostly used in low-calorie foods to provide sweetness but with lesser calories. You can use xylitol in home baking as a substitute for regular white sugar (in the ratio 1:1) although the browning won't be as much and also not that you cannot use it were yeast is used as the raising agent.

How to effectively cut down on your sugar intake

Making a few tweaks in your diet will help you cut down on unnecessary junk and sugar consumption.

1. Stay away from diet foods that are low fat as they tend to have high sugar levels; you should instead have the regular versions in small portions.
2. Balance your intake of carbs with protein, fruits and veggies. Protein foods like fish, turkey and kitchen are lean and slow down stomach emptying. Fruits and veggies are high in fiber which takes longer to digest, keeping you full longer.
3. Cut down the sugar you add to hot beverages such as hot chocolate and cappuccinos. Instead of adding 2 teaspoons of sugar to you hot chocolate, add a teaspoon of sugar and half a teaspoon of cinnamon.

Cinnamon stabilizes the blood sugar levels and also adds a punch of flavor without all the unnecessary sweetness of sugar.

4. Stay away from foods that claim to be 'sugar free', in most cases these foods contain synthetic sweeteners such as sucralose, aspartame and saccharine. These sweeteners send confusing messages to your brain causing you to overeat.

5. When making your own recipes, reduce the sugar indicated and increase the amount of spices recommended to boost the taste and flavor.

6. Swap refined grain products such as white bread, pasta and rice for whole grain versions which have a higher fiber content keeping you full longer.

7. For a pick me up, have a handful of nuts, a piece of fruit or a small tub of pain yogurt that all have protein which helps balance your blood sugar levels and energy levels.

8. Swap fruit juices for smoothies that contain all the fiber from the fruit therein keeping you full longer. Stay away from processed soft drinks and alcohols which have hidden sugars

Is food addiction real?

Most of us if not all of us can attest to having a love-hate relationship with our food at one point in time. This usually stems from feelings of guilt and shame especially after eating a whole box of cookies, chocolates, donuts or any other food/ snack. The pleasure of over-indulging in our favorite food is followed almost immediately by feelings of shame for not being able to stop ourselves say after two cookies and this wretched feeling leads us to eat more and more.

Being addicted to sugar does not mean that you have zero willpower or that you have an emotional eating disorder. It is purely biological and it is driven by neurotransmitters and hormones that fuel the sugar cravings that in turn lead you to over-eat. This is the reason why over 40% of our children are overweight and why approximately 70% of adults are overweight.

Is a sugar detox necessary?

Do you wake up feeling like you are just from running a marathon instead of having a good night's rest, or are you constantly fatigued even when you haven't done any energy intensive activity? Well, this is a sure sign that your body is not getting all the essentials nutrients to ensure that all your organs and physiological processes are running smoothly. We eat foods that are laden with sugar and have very little nutritional value.

To reverse this, a sugar detox is necessary to deliver us from the enslaving addictive cycle of sugar cravings and overeating that is slowly robbing us of our health. First, it is important to note that there is nothing wrong with your willpower, what we need is science to break this vicious cycle. But, don't fret; we are not going to be taking a pure soup diet or any bland or boring foods.

Step 1: Make a conscious decision

Our bodies are more self-sufficient than we give them credit for and when it's time for you to embark on a sugar detox, you can rely on your body to tell you exactly that. There are three things that you will need to watch out for by answering the following questions:

Pre-diabesity

Do you crave sugar all the time? Are you overweight? Do you have diabetes or are you pre-diabetic? Do you have lots of trouble trying to lose weight? Do you have high cholesterol levels? Do you have belly fat?

Food addiction

Do you find yourself eating even when you are not hungry? Do you feel extremely bad after eating certain foods? Do you avoid certain activities because of your eating habits? Do you get withdrawal symptoms if you cut back on sugar or some of your favorite snacks? Do you have an uncontrollable need for more and more of the same 'bad foods' just to feel better especially after something bad happens to you?

Feeling like crap!

Do you experience bloating, reflux, joint and muscle pain, brain fog, allergies, irritable bowel, mood issues and more?

If you answer positively for any of the above questions, it is a sure sign of a cry for help from your body and it's a clear indication that you need a sugar detox.

Step 2: Go cold turkey for 10 days

The one sure way to handle a physiological addiction is to stop it immediately! Addicts who go to rehab are not allowed to have one more drink or one more line of cocaine. Considering sugar is eight times as addictive as cocaine, the same rule of immediate cessation should apply. The key is to stop consuming all forms of sugar, artificial sweeteners and processed food products – which cause supercharged cravings and a dragging metabolism leading to fat storage.

Additionally, lookout for anything that has hydrogenated fats, Trans fats or MSG. ideally, for the next 10 days, you should refrain from eating anything that comes in a can, box or package. Go for natural and real fresh food.

Step 3: No liquid calories

Liquids are digested faster than solid food and so if you are taking sugar laden drinks they are going to be digested faster making you hungry and craving for some more. Before you know it, you will have exceeded your recommended daily intake which will not only make you fat but sick. A single can of soda increases a child's chance of being overweight and obese by 60% and a woman's chance of getting type 2 diabetes by 80% so stay as far away as possible!

Step 4: Protein power

Having protein at every meal especially at breakfast is one of the best ways to balance insulin and blood sugar and also reduce the cravings because they take long to digest thus keeping you full up to your next meal.

Include eggs, wild caught fish, nuts and seeds, chicken, whole grains and lean meats in all your meals.

Step 5: Eat all the veggies you want!

Vegetable are endowed with healthy carbs, fiber vitamins, minerals and a dose of protein. You can eat as much as you want without having to worry about damaging your health but you have to focus more on non-starch vegetables. Dark leafy greens, broccoli, cauliflower, asparagus, mushrooms, zucchini, onions, tomatoes, fennel, artichokes, eggplant, green beans, okra, etc.

Step 6: Go for healthy fats

Healthy fats don't make you fat, sugar does! Fats fuel your cells, keep you full longer and balance your blood sugar levels. Olive oil, avocado, coconut products, nuts and seeds and wild caught fish are very good source of healthy fats.

Step 7: Always have an emergency pack

The worst thing that can happen as you try to get away from sugar is find yourself surrounded by maze of fast food joints and convenience stores when your glucose levels are dropping fast. You should always have a small pack of healthy ingredients made from healthy fats and protein. Fresh berries, nut butters, salmon jerky, nuts and seeds are some of the ready-to-go snacks you can always carry in your handbag or backpack.

Step 8: breathe when in distress

When faced with stressful situations your hormones literally go haywire. Your cortisol levels shoot through the roof which make you really hungry and in such situations, a bowl of baby carrot is not the first thing you reach out for. The best thing to do in such a situation is take very deep breathes. This may sound ridiculous but it actually activates the vagus nerve, which switches your metabolism from storing fat to burning fat.

Stay calm and take 5 very slow and deep breathes and you will start feeling better.

Step 9: Tackle inflammation

Inflammation is the number one culprit behind all chronic illnesses. Sugar, Trans fats and flour are the three main drivers of food sensitivity that leads to inflammation. The problem is we always crave for what's bad for us. For this 10 days, quit sugar and all processed foods and about four days into the detox you are going to experience new found energy than anything you have experienced before.

Step 10: Nothing beats beauty sleep

You have probably noticed that you eat more the next day if you don't get enough sleep. This is because, your body recovers from all the day's strenuous activities during sleep and this is also the time the repair of damaged cells occurs. When you don't get enough sleep, the brain triggers the release of two hormones, adrenalin – to provide you with energy though out the day and cortisol – to ensure that this energy is constantly replenished by inducing hunger.

In the end you eat more than your body needs and because not all the energy is used up, you end up storing all the excess as fat. Aim at sleeping for a minimum of 7 hours every.

These ten steps will help rewire your system and stop the cravings that can leave you feeling crippled and helpless.

The key to fighting addiction to sugar is to tame your brain and to teach it that you can function optimally without unhealthy sugars. You may never have deemed it possible to crave an apple in place of a snickers bar but take this detox challenge and you will be pleasantly surprised. We are now going to look at some yummy sugar free recipes that are to die for!

Recipes

1. Fluffy Sugar Free, Gluten Free Pancakes

Ingredients

- 1 cup rice flour
- 4 tsp buttermilk powder
- 3 tbsp tapioca flour
- 1 ½ tsp baking power
- 1/3 cup potato starch
- 2eggs
- ½ tsp xantham gum
- ½ tsp baking soda
- 3 tsp canola oil
- ½ tsp salt
- 1 pkt natural sugar substitute
- 2 cups water

Directions

Combine all the dry ingredients in a bowl then stir in the eggs and water until well blended then add the oil. Continue beating until you are left with very few lumps.

Now place a non-stick skillet over medium heat and lightly coat the skillet with cooking spray. You can alternatively use a griddle, if you prefer.

Use a ladle to spoon the batter onto your skillet/ griddle and cook until you start seeing bubbles form. Flip the pancake and cook the other side until golden.

Serve with fresh berries. Enjoy!

2. Peanut Butter Grilled Pork

Ingredients

- 2 pcs pork tenderloin, fat trimmed off
- 1 tsp smooth and natural peanut butter
- 1 clove garlic, minced
- 1 tbsp fresh ginger, finely grated
- 3 tsp soy sauce
- 1 tbsp sesame oil
- 1 tsp natural honey
- Salt to taste

Directions

Combine soy sauce, sesame oil, honey, peanut butter, curry powder, ginger, garlic and salt in a mixing bowl until well blended. Place the pork in a zip lock plastic bag then pour in the marinade. Toss well to coat the tenderloins evenly, press out the air then seal the bag and chill in you fridge overnight.

An outdoor grill is perfect for this recipe so preheat your outdoor grill at high heat.

Meanwhile, remove the pork from the plastic bag and pat excess marinade using a paper towel. Leave the pork to sit at room temperature as the grill is heating up.

Lightly coat the grill grate using cooking spray and cook the pork for about 3 minutes per side until cooked to desire. Once ready, remove the pork from the grill and loosely cover using kitchen foil for 5 minutes and then you can serve. Enjoy!

3. French Toast Casserole

Ingredients

- 5 cups cubed sugar free bread
- 1 ½ cups milk
- 4 eggs
- 2 tsp ground cinnamon
- Stevia to taste
- 1 tsp vanilla extract
- Olive oil cooking spray

Directions

Coat a rectangular baking dish with cooking spray.

Arrange the bread cubes at the bottom of the prepared baking dish. Now beat the eggs milk, 1 teaspoon cinnamon, 1 tablespoon stevia and vanilla extract in a bowl until frothy then pour over the bread cubes.

For best results, refrigerate overnight.

Preheat your oven to 350^0F.

When ready to cook, combine the remaining cinnamon with two teaspoons stevia and gently sprinkle over the casserole.

Bake for about 40 minute until the top is golden and crunchy.

Remove from oven and let stand for 10 minutes before serving.

Enjoy!

4. Simple And Quick Grilled Cheese

Ingredients

- 2 slices cheddar cheese, sharp
- 1 tbsp softened butter
- 2 slices whole grain sugar fee bread
- 1 tsp fresh basil, finely chopped
- 1 tbsp fresh parsley, finely chopped
- 1 tsp fresh rosemary finely chopped
- 1 tsp fresh dill, finely chopped
- 1 tsp oregano

Directions

Spread the butter on one side for each slice of bread and place a slice of cheddar on the unbuttered side of one slice of bread. Sprinkle the herbs on the other slice of bread on the unbuttered side.

Now sandwich the two filled slices. Place a skillet on medium heat and once hot gently place the sandwich on the hot skillet. Cook each buttered side for about 3 minute until golden and crisp and the cheese melts. Enjoy!

5. Creamy And Nutty Pineapple Pudding

Ingredients

- 1 can unsweetened pineapple chunks, crushed and undrained
- 1 package instant pistachio pudding ix, unsweetened
- 1 pkt vanilla flavored yogurt, sugar free
- 1 pkt plain yogurt
- 1 cup whipped topping, unsweetened

Directions

Combine the crushed pineapple, pistachio mix, and the two yogurts in a glass bowl until smooth. Use a rubber spatula to gently fold in the whipped topping. Cover using plastic wrap and chill in the fridge for a minimum of 2 hours. Enjoy!

6. Un-Sugared Rugelach

Ingredients

- 2 ¾ cups all-purpose flour
- 1 cup margarine
- 1 cup walnuts, chopped
- 1 cup softened apricot spreadable fruit, unsweetened
- 1 cup raisins, chopped
- 25g softened cream cheese
- 2 tsp vanilla extract

Directions

Use an electric mixer to cream the margarine and cream cheese. Next add the vanilla followed by the flour. Cover the bowl with cling wrap and chill the dough.

Meanwhile, prepare the filling by combining the walnuts, raisins and cinnamon in a food processor by making short pulses in order to chop and not grind the nuts and raisins.

Divide the dough into four and roll out the four portions to form circles. Sprinkle the filing on top of the circles about ¼ cup for ach circle.

Use a cookie cutter to cut out 16 wedges from each circle. Roll each wedge from the base to the tip and place down on baking sheets lined with parchment paper.

Bake for about 15 minutes at 375^0F until golden. Remove from oven and transfer to a cooling rack to cool. Enjoy!

Don't Be Part Of The Statistic! (Conclusion)

Having concrete information on sugar puts you in the driver's seat and all that is required of you is to floor the pedal to the metal in the journey of securing your health. As a general rule, a healthy diet is one that is high in healthy fats and extremely low in sugar and any non-vegetable carbs and that has a moderate and healthy amount of good quality protein from lean meats and whole grains and legumes.

Your health comes first, make the right decision!

I want you to thank yourself for wanting to change and I hope you walk away inspired or smarter.

As you read on you will find tips used by entrepreneurs, and motivational thoughts that come from coaches and entrepreneurs themselves. Have Fun and good luck with your endeavors. Before moving on, I just want to remind you that we are all born on this earth as equals. Some may have more support than others, but we can only characterize ourselves by our own actions. In other words, everyone in this world has potential hidden in a box. Some choose to find a way to open it, and some just leave it there.

Think about this and try to figure out who you are.

Some may be okay living an average life, but then there are also others who constantly look for better.

Life Hacking Tips Used by the Entrepreneurs!

Coffee Nap

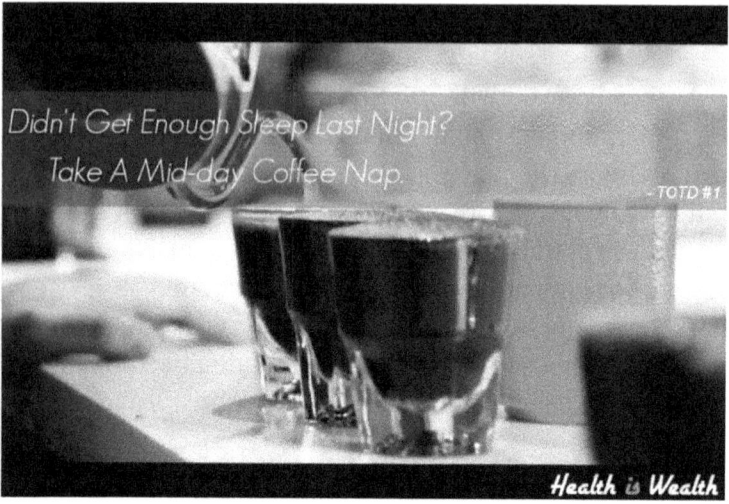

This method provided is called, "Caffeine Nap", where you drink a cup of coffee and nap for 15 minutes. The 15 minutes gives you time to rest and allows the caffeine to travel through your gastro-intestinal tract. This will provide you with a refreshing reboot by the time you wake up. But don't go over the 15-20 minutes limit or else you'll wake up in a sleepy state.

Plan the Night Before

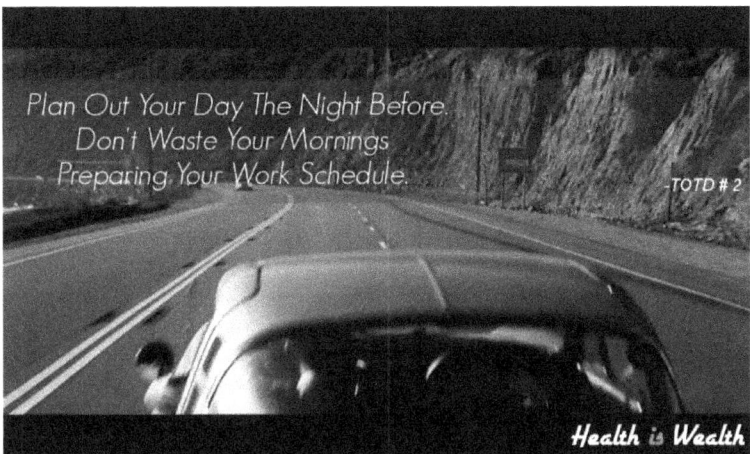

Plan Out Your Day The Night Before.
Don't Waste Your Mornings
Preparing Your Work Schedule.

-TOTD # 2

Health is Wealth

You heard of this before, you can either work hard or work smart. It's your choice. There's nothing wrong about working hard, but what's the point of working hard if the results are not there. You need to work smart and change up your routine so that your work is actually effective. Tonight before you go to bed, plan out your work for the next day so that you don't waste time in the morning. Don't waste your mornings on planning out what you want to work on as you are wasting your brains fuel. Your brain is packed with fuel from last night's rest, so go use it on something productive. Don't be like the majority of people who sit on their desk wondering what they need to do. Hope this helps!

Acknowledge Your Accomplishments, But....

You have one win in your hand, but that's not enough. It's not time to celebrate just yet. This is only a small win towards your goal. If you celebrate now, you might just lose the fire that you've always had in you to pursue your dreams. So when you reach a goal, recognize it. Please do so as it will be your source of motivation. The motivation that tells you, maybe it is possible. Maybe this dream isn't out of my reach. Just remember to set your goals high and when you do reach them, set them even higher the next time.

Must Always Take a Break

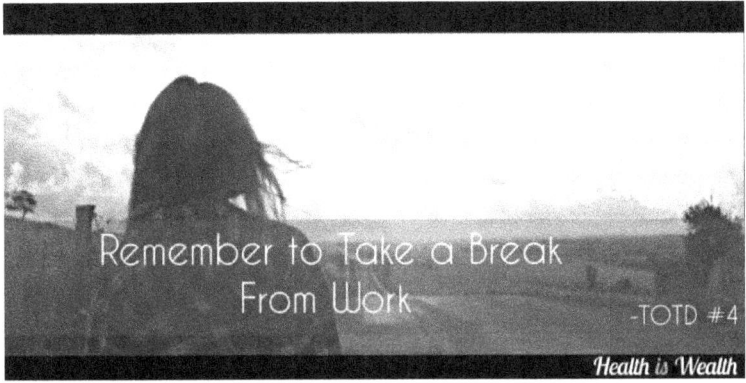

Most of us work for a living, and sometimes we work so hard that we feel too tired to spend time with the people we love. Just remember that our work will always change, but our family will always be there. On another thought, we need to take breaks during excessive periods of work, so that we can replenish our thoughts. Take a walk and get some fresh air.

Are You Committed?

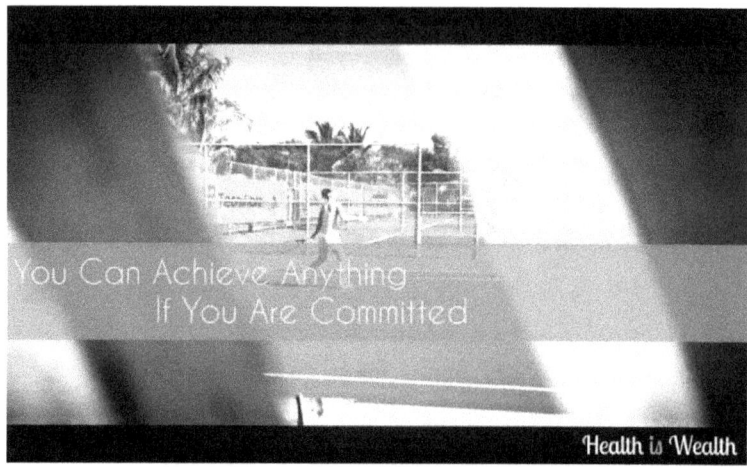

Are you interested or are you committed to achieving your current goals? Most may ask, what is the difference? If you have interest in fulfilling your goals, then you will complete your task and never look back. In other words, you will do things the same way as how most people do it. However, if you are committed to your situation, then you will find yourself working more than you need to, and trying to improve your current goals, although they are already good enough. Successful entrepreneurs are successful because they have a purpose behind their tasks, it is more than just interest. So just ask yourself, are you interested or are you committed to what you are currently doing.

There Should Never Be a Plan "B"

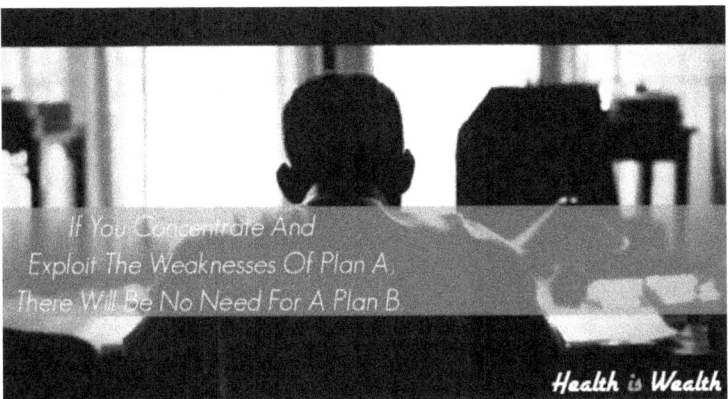

You've all heard of Plan B's. They are there to back you up just in case Plan A doesn't work. But what's the point of spending half your time on Plan A and half your time on Plan B. Instead, use your time to focus solely on Plan A so that you can perfect it. A perfect plan is better than two average plans. I've always grown up being told "If you do it right the first time, you won't have to do it a second time". So why do it a second time, you're just wasting energy. Perfect your 1st attempt so that you can move on and accomplish other things in life.

Become a Warrior

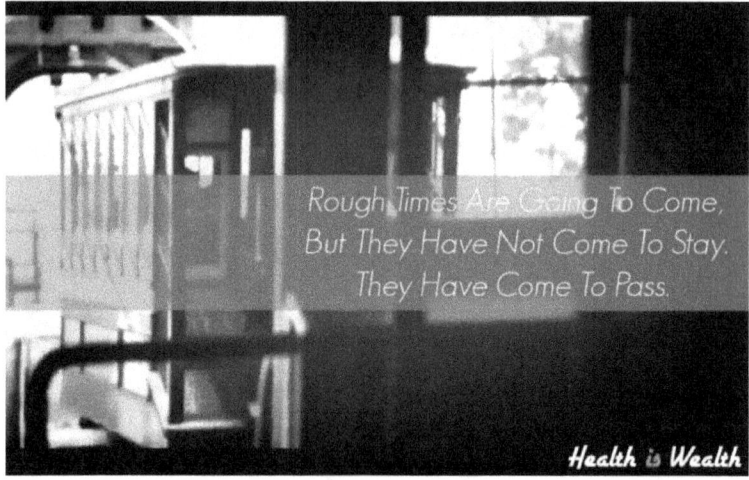

Rough Times Are Going To Come,
But They Have Not Come To Stay.
They Have Come To Pass.

Health is Wealth

It's not like we're never going to get hurt in life. And it's not like these episodes are meant to devastate us. These harsh times are just the flow of life and everyone gets them, we just need to do our part and accept them. It may sound easy but it really isn't. To accept tragedy or a mishap in your life is going to be hard because we're humans. We're emotional and that's understandable, but what about life. Life isn't going to wait for you, it's like a train with no brakes. The Sun is still going to shine, and the Moon is still going to glow. So try not to mourn for too long. These hard times are bound to come, but they have not come to stay. They have come to pass.

A Forgotten Lifestyle

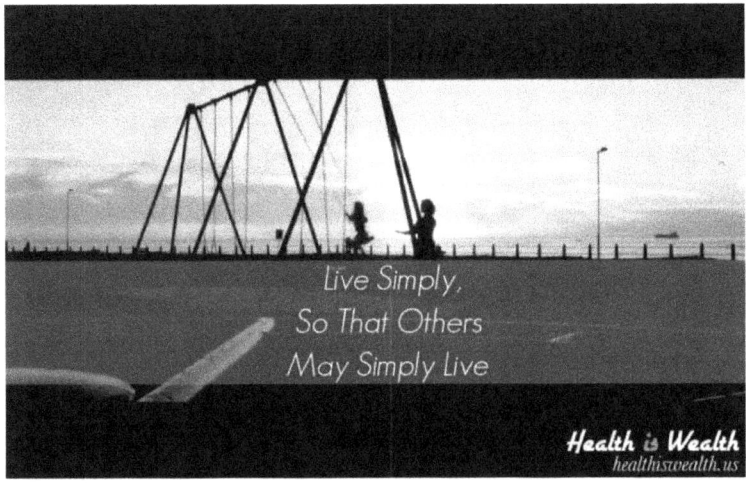

*Live Simply,
So That Others
May Simply Live*

Health is Wealth
healthiswealth.us

This is probably going to be my favorite for a while. Live simply, so that others may simply live. A simple saying that would do wonders for the world. In a world where capitalism is King, we often get carried away by lavish lifestyles that we envy of others. There's nothing wrong with treating yourself after a hard day's work. It's just that sometimes we become a bit too selfish. There are many people around us that aren't even able to even eat 3 times a day, and here we are complaining about getting the newest gadgets. Our job to live simply is not going to kill us. We may miss out on getting a few designer handbags or suits, but at the end of the day those funds will allow the unfortunate to live another day.

Stop Waiting and Just Do It

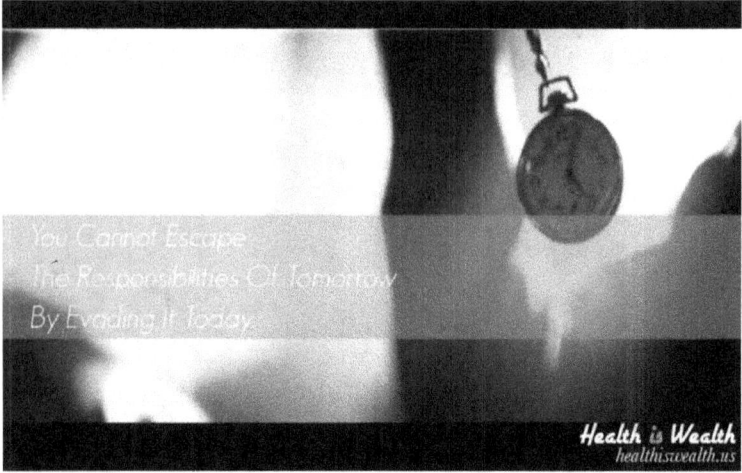

I'll do it later. For some reason we only feel obliged to start working when the deadline is near. Maybe you just need pressure to start working. We all put off work until later and our work becomes faulty when we're done. No time left to correct your mistakes. But that's not how successful people succeed and we need to instill in our minds to organize your workload so that you don't do last minute work.

You Are Only One Person, But...

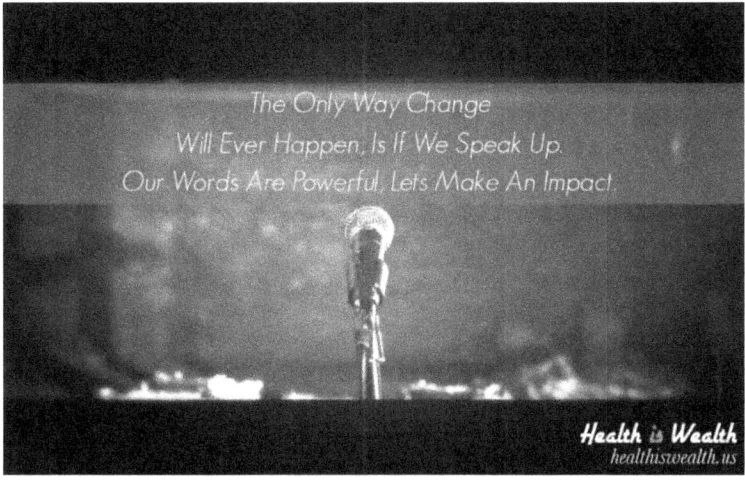

The Only Way Change
Will Ever Happen, Is If We Speak Up.
Our Words Are Powerful, Lets Make An Impact.

Health is Wealth
healthiswealth.us

This was always my problem. I'm guilty of the, "but I'm just one person" crime. I'm so used to assuming that other people are going to make an effort to change their surroundings that I suppose my input wouldn't make a difference. So what if you're just one person. If you're making a change and people around you see it, then they'll be inspired to make the change with you. You are never just one. There may be many others in the room who have the same idea as you, but are not confident enough to share. Stand up and speak your mind so that confidence may grow in them too. The only way change will ever happen, is if we speak up. Our words are powerful, let's make an impact. Don't ever think of yourself as just one.

My Dream Never Faded. Your Doubts Just made it More Clear to Me

They Asked Him, How Did He Do It?
He Replied,
There Was No One Here
To Tell Me I Couldn't Do It

Health is Wealth

Are you sure? No one has ever done it before, so how will you do it? It's Impossible.

Well that's not new. People telling you what's possible and what's impossible. But what do they know. They don't know how much time and effort you put in every day and night into your work. If they tell you that it's impossible, let it fuel your fire. Proving people wrong was always a hobby of mine. So go out there and work. And when that day comes, you could tell your doubters that it was always possible.

Even if no one sees it for you, you must see it for yourself. And just like that you are on the road to success.

How's Your Willpower?

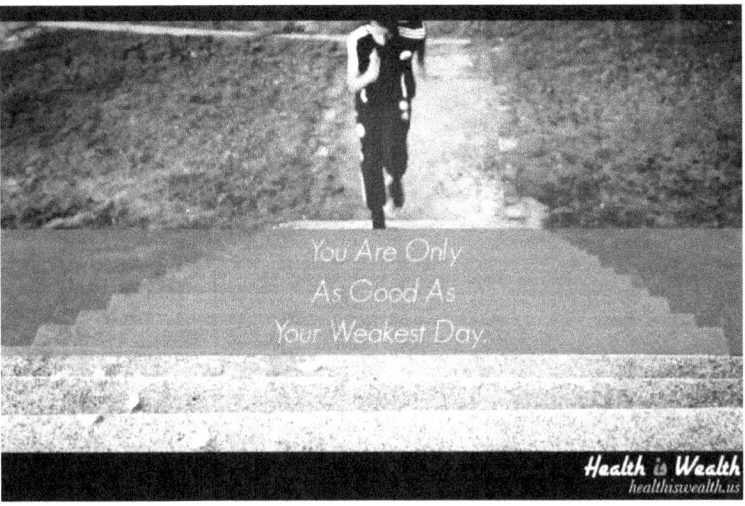

Stop setting goals and stopping half way. Sometimes we get inspired and decide to dream big. And after the next day the inspiration is gone and we decide to quit. The problem is not that we have set your goals too high. There's no such thing as setting your goals too high. The problem is us. If we don't want it bad enough, then we will be like the majority of people who start something and then say it's getting nowhere. Well don't expect results to come in just a couple of days, this is a long term commitment. We have to be committed to what we do in order to get far. We can start and end half way, but what does that really say about our willpower. You are only as good as your weakest day.

We Used to Dream a Lot

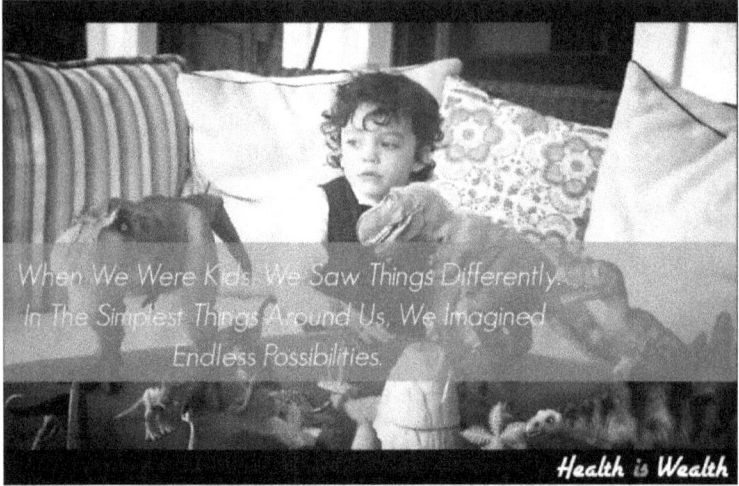

When We Were Kids, We Saw Things Differently. In The Simplest Things Around Us, We Imagined Endless Possibilities.

Health is Wealth

Back then we used to tie a towel around our neck and jump off our beds only to soar for a couple of seconds. But those couple of seconds were enough to allow us to feel like superheroes. We turned that towel into a cape and it gave us an identity. When we were kids, we saw things differently. In the simplest things around us, we imagined endless possibilities. Who would have known that a chunk of metal would help us fly around the world? That's absurd right? It's hard to imagine an airplane from looking at a chunk of metal. As we grow older we slowly push our imaginations aside, and that towel that used to help us fly is just a rag to us now. We've grown up in a world filled with pessimists, whom only know how to provide doubts into our imaginations. It's hard to be innovative when we have so much doubts in our own ideas. So just let those imaginations come back and give them another chance. You'll never know where those imaginations will take you.

G.R.I.N.D.

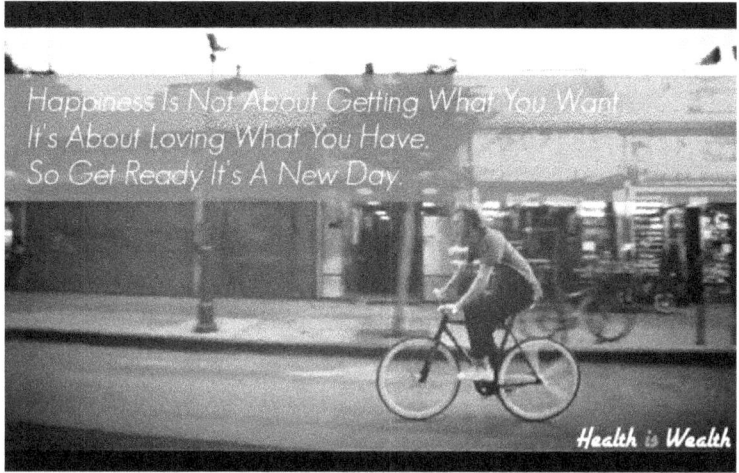

Happiness Is Not About Getting What You Want
It's About Loving What You Have.
So Get Ready It's A New Day.

Health is Wealth

Sometimes I feel like I'm not making any progress toward my goals and it frightens me. My dreams and goals are still there, but I have my doubts like any human would. So today I turned on my speakers and Asher Roth was on. It was only then that I realized that I was doing it all wrong. My goal was to work hard so that I could buy my parents stuff that they would be happy to have. I wanted them to be happy. I wanted them to know that in the near future, their working hours would be lessened and that I would bombard them with gifts.

But it wasn't until today, that I realize how faulty my goals were. I was so focused on spending time on work for a better future that I nearly forgot about spending time with my parents in the present. Spending money on my parents can come a little later, but for now it's about spending time with the people you love. Happiness isn't not about getting what you want all the time, it's about loving what you have. So get ready, it's a new day.

Appreciate What You Have!

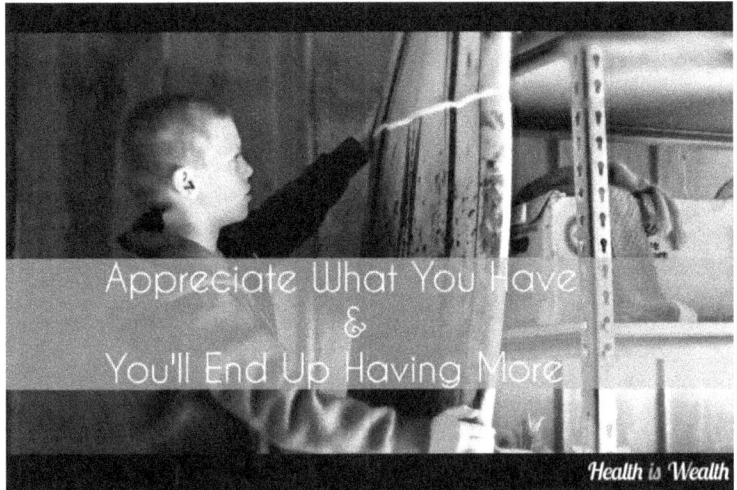

Today we are so focused with getting new things that we neglect what we already have. We look forward to creating new relationships, and leave behind the relationships we already have. Instead of trying to fix the problems in our current situations, we look for something new as a solution, but at the end of the day we are just dragging out the problem. So let's fix something today, before looking elsewhere. When a friendship is confronted with problems, they settle the problem with each other and grow stronger together.

Stuck in Your Comfort Zone?

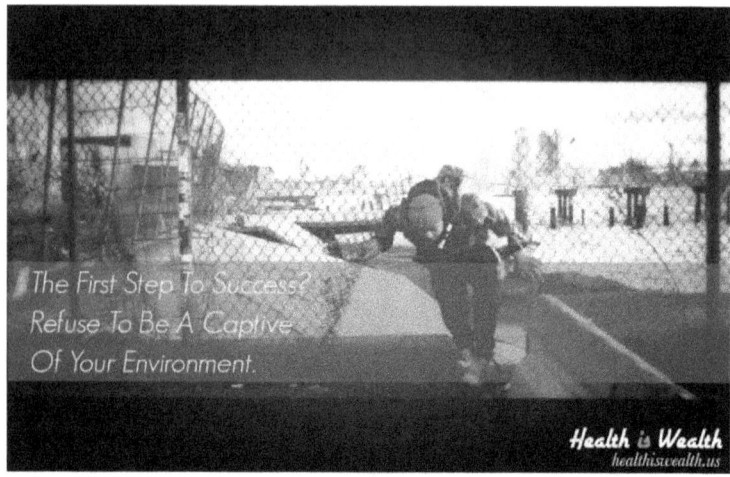

The First Step To Success?
Refuse To Be A Captive
Of Your Environment.

Health is Wealth
healthiswealth.us

You say you want to be healthy. You say you want to be rich. But are you doing anything towards these goals. Surrounding yourself with a room full of junk food is not going to help. Neither is hanging around people who don't believe in working hard. You need to get out of your old environment and go find a new one. Stop being trapped in the misery that is around you. Go meet new friends that actually care about the wellness of their body and people who set new goals every week. Once you are in their environment, you'll find yourself trying to work as hard as or even harder than them. Place yourself in a healthy environment, but first you have to leave your old one.

Thank you for taking the time to read this book and may you always have a perfectly balanced life. If you haven't already read my author's description before purchasing this book, you would know that I am also the founder of Finicky. The images provided by the book come from my website, "Finicky.us"

Preview of "Public Speaking: 7 Essentials Steps Used by Top Entrepreneurs"

You may purchase this book by <u>clicking here</u>

Or by using this link <u>http://amzn.to/1dsxVg9</u>

The feeling of nervousness or stage-fright when presenting to an audience is perfectly normal. Even the best public speakers still get nervous. This is a part of being human, we are wired to be worried about our reputation and public speaking is a threat to us. In psychological terms, our fight or flight responses comes into play and our body starts feeling different.

Before I go on any further, I would just like to tell you that the fears of public speaking are not to be overcome, we need to adapt to our public speaking environment. I would like you to keep this in mind as you continue to read on.

Before considering talking in public there are some things you must be aware of. The first thing you should do before speaking in public is to find out who you are and what you need.

The feedback you will receive after speaking in public is relevant for what you are going to do next. You should always meditate and answer these questions: Who am I? What do I want? What do I need?